I would like to thank Dr Richard Ban_____ _____chael Neill, Dr Roger Callahan, Paul Duddridge, _____ _____taples, Dr Hugh Willbourn, Michael Breen, _____ _____oung and Mike Osborne.

I would also like to thank all o_____ _____rticipants at my weight-loss seminars who hav_____ _____ed me develop this system.

Also by Paul McKenna

HOW TO MEND YOUR BROKEN HEART
(with Hugh Willbourn)

THE HYPNOTIC WORLD OF PAUL McKENNA

CHANGE YOUR LIFE IN SEVEN DAYS

I CAN MAKE YOU THIN

•

PAUL McKENNA Ph.D.

Edited by Michael Neill

BANTAM PRESS

LONDON • TORONTO • SYDNEY • AUCKLAND • JOHANNESBURG

TRANSWORLD PUBLISHERS
61-63 Uxbridge Road, London W5 5SA
a division of The Random House Group Ltd

RANDOM HOUSE AUSTRALIA (PTY) LTD
20 Alfred Street, Milsons Point, Sydney,
New South Wales 2061, Australia

RANDOM HOUSE NEW ZEALAND LTD
18 Poland Road, Glenfield, Auckland 10, New Zealand

RANDOM HOUSE SOUTH AFRICA (PTY) LTD
Endulini, 5a Jubilee Road, Parktown 2193, South Africa

Published 2005 by Bantam Press
a division of Transworld Publishers

A catalogue record for this book is available
from the British Library.
ISBN 0593 05054 1

Typeset in 11/16 pt Palatino
by Falcon Oast Graphic Art Ltd.

Printed and bound in Great Britain by Clays Ltd, Bungay, Suffolk

5 7 9 10 8 6 4

Papers used by Transworld Publishers are natural, recyclable products
made from wood grown in sustainable forests. The manufacturing processes conform to the
environmental regulations of the country of origin.

The Weight-Loss Mind-Programming CD

Your mind is like a computer – it has its own software which helps you to organize your thinking and behaviour. Having worked with all sorts of people with different problems over many years, I have learned that almost all problems stem from the same cause – negative programmes running in the unconscious mind.

This book comes with a powerful mind-programming CD that will fill your unconscious mind with positive willpower. While you become absorbed in to a natural state of relaxation, I will reprogramme your computer – your unconscious mind – so that you will change the way that you think about food and feel better about yourself. I will give you suggestions that will help you to change your behaviour, eat better, speed up your metabolism and escape from the fixation with food.

It's best to listen to it when you have about half an hour where you can safely relax completely. As you listen to it regularly, you will re-enforce all the changes you are making. In fact, it will make it much easier to stick to the golden rules I share with you in this book.

The latest research into the effectiveness of these and similar techniques has shown that listening to this CD over and over again, every day, will dramatically enhance your ability to lose weight. You don't have to believe it, only use it!

WARNING:

DO NOT LISTEN TO THE CD WHILE DRIVING OR OPERATING HEAVY MACHINERY OR IF YOU SUFFER FROM EPILEPSY OR CLINICAL DEPRESSION. IF IN DOUBT, CONSULT YOUR DOCTOR.

CONTENTS

PREFACE

As a medical nutritionist for more than two decades, I have seen patients lose weight on any number of diet programmes, then watched as they struggled to maintain their weight loss. The ability of overweight individuals to accept chronic food deprivation at levels as low as 400 calories a day for extended periods of time has never ceased to amaze me. Nor has the sad reality that most of them regain their hard-won losses. A significant number have undergone this process repeatedly.

Why couldn't obese individuals stay on a diet? Over the years, some patients told me that they just couldn't stop themselves. Others said they just ate mindlessly, often not knowing what they were eating. The common belief that eating is controllable has led us to expect people 'to behave' or pay the price of public shame. But diets don't work, eating is not due to lack of will-power. Eating, ultimately, is under the control of the brain.

In our world, where food is freely available, maintaining weight loss by dieting requires a continuous conscious effort to eat less. Like our inability to resist sleep, our brains will override our minds and make us eat. This is in the nature of any living organism where the brain dictates behaviour.

How can we alter this course? The answer lies not in the diet but in changing our response to signals from the brain. That is behaviour modification. In this book are the keys to accomplishing that which seems impossible: losing weight and keeping it off.

No fad diets recommended here, rather an approach to controlling the response to hunger and, even more importantly, a way of altering the appetitive drive by reducing the stress that dieting causes.

This is a revolutionary approach and it is the only approach that will be successful long term without the use of medication. I recommend that the reader keep an open mind and closely follow the expert advice given here. This approach requires work, but in persistence will lie victory for those who have long fought this battle.

Ronald Ruden, M.D., Ph.D.
Lenox Hill Hospital
New York
Author of *The Craving Brain*

AN IMPORTANT NOTE FROM PAUL McKENNA

How would you like to eat whatever you want whenever you want and still lose weight?

I know that seems like an outrageous claim, and it's true.

This system is so simple you will probably find it difficult at first to believe that it will work. That's because you have been brainwashed by diets to believe that weight loss is difficult, and it's not. In fact, an independent research study into the effectiveness of my system showed that the system you are about to learn is seven times more successful than any diet!

Recently I met a lady who had attended one of my seminars and lost a considerable amount of weight. She told me that she was angry. When I asked her why, she said it was because she had spent years torturing herself with diets and feeling like a failure. In fact, she'd added up all the money she'd spent on diets, weight-loss programmes and special foods and it came to thousands of pounds. If only she'd known how easy weight loss really is.

Some of what I am about to say will fly in the face of what you've done in the past and what you think is 'right'. You've tried other methods of weight loss and they didn't work or they only worked temporarily.

No matter what you've tried before, it's time to do something radically different.

The exact same approach that I am about to share with you has helped thousands and thousands of people to lose weight easily and feel significantly better about themselves. Now it's your turn . . .

To your good health,
Paul McKenna

CHAPTER ONE

•

Are You Ready for Something Truly Different?

Are you ready for something truly different?

This may well be the shortest book on losing weight you have ever read. But don't be fooled by its size. As I think you'll agree, thin is good, and it's what's inside that really matters.

I've worked hard to get this little book as concise as possible – so concise that you can probably finish the whole thing in less than a day. But what a day it will be!

During that time, you will not only discover what's been keeping you from the body you desire, but you'll also learn the simplest and most effective weight-loss system ever devised. It's a system that has helped people who felt as though they had

> *'I am delighted I feel more in control of my life. I no longer live to eat, I eat to live.'*
>
> JANET ALLEN, ADMINISTRATOR

failed at every diet in the world, or been overweight all their lives, as well as those people who just wanted to lose weight and feel great for life.

Whether your primary goal is to lose weight, lead a healthier lifestyle, feel really happy with your body, or just to be able to shift those last ten pounds, then this system is exactly what you've been looking for!

I'll also reveal the truth about exercise and share with you some simple but powerful techniques to supercharge your metabolism, control your cravings, and let go of the emotional issues you used to stuff down with food. Finally, I'll teach you some of my favourite mind-programming techniques, which you can use to feel better now and in the future; you'll be able to put on the CD any time you want to reinforce the principles deep into your unconscious mind.

But don't take my word for it – just follow my instructions step by step and notice how your body, and life, begin to change for the better.

Learning the secrets of naturally thin people

Throughout the book, I will share with you the secrets that I have gleaned by studying naturally thin people. These are not the stick-figure models whose waif-like physiques come from eating disorders, drug addiction and airbrushing, but rather those people in life who somehow seem to be able to eat whatever they want and stay slim.

By developing the eating habits of naturally thin people, you'll be able to eat anything you want, whenever you want and still lose weight. Let's face it – you can have what you want, or you can have your reasons for not having it. So, if *absolutely anyone can lose weight with this system*, the only other question we need to ask is this:

Why aren't you thin yet?

There are three main patterns I have observed that keep people from living happily at their desired weight. As you read through the descriptions below, notice which of these apply to you. Then, when we begin re-programming your mind in Chapter Three, you will be able to apply just the right tools and begin to lose weight immediately . . .

Pattern One: Obsessive Dieting

I was browsing through some of the recent releases in the weight-loss section of my local bookshop. What I found astounding was that despite the fact that nearly all of them were filled with 'forbidden food' lists, menus and calorie guides, they each began with the words 'This is NOT a diet'.

Let's begin by getting one thing straight:

A diet is any system of eating that attempts to exert external control over what, where, when or how much you eat.

Dieting has got a bad name over the past few years, and there's a good reason for that – scientific research shows that more than 90 per cent of people who attempt to lose weight by dieting fail.

Whenever somebody comes up to tell me about the weight they've lost on this great new diet, I ask them to come back and tell me about it in six months' time. If they are still happy about their weight and their diet in six months I am ready to listen. Unfortunately, I am still waiting for anybody to come back.

My theory? Too many diets, too few results. With over 25,000 diet books currently in print, many of which contain directly contradictory information, is it any wonder you find yourself as confused and misguided as the multi-billion-dollar weight-loss industry?

> 'Paul McKenna's weight-loss system is the best thing I have ever done.'
>
> PETER WILKINSON, DESIGNER

It's not just that diets don't work, many of them are an outright con. In fact, when I see celebrities who have 'battled their weight problems' endorsing the latest fad diet, I don't know how they keep a straight face. In most instances, what they have actually done is tried a diet, lost weight, and then put the weight back on again a few months later. Then they simply tried another diet, lost weight, and promoted that one for a few months until the weight started piling back on.

In case you haven't picked up on the message here, it's this:

Forget about dieting. For ever. Diets are no more than training courses in how to get fat and feel like a failure.

The more diets people try and fail at the more they convince themselves that they will never be able to lose weight. What nobody tells you is that the real reason most weight-loss programmes don't work is nothing to do with you – it's to do with human biology.

In his seminal study into human starvation during the Second World War, biological researcher Ancel Keyes discovered that reducing people's diet to a state of semi-starvation produced symptoms of irritability, loss of endurance and obsessive behaviour around food, including but not limited to lying, hoarding and stealing.

Even more telling, in the three-month period after the semi-starvation was ended and people could once again eat whatever they wanted, their obsession with food continued. Many people ate up to eight times as much food as they had done before the study began. (Does any of this sound familiar?)

That experiment, documented in the 1950s treatise *The Biology of Human Starvation*, is considered unreplicable. After all, to purposely starve people would be cruel and inhumane. But here's an interesting fact: the semi-starvation rations from the original study amounted to about 1,500 calories a day – more than is allowed in any number of the thousands of diets currently in vogue.

What all this goes to show is that depriving yourself of food is the worst possible way to lose weight. And if what you're doing isn't working, you need to do something different.

Pattern Two: Emotional Eating

I am convinced that after diets, emotional eating is the number-one cause of obesity in the world. Many times people eat because they are bored, or lonely or miserable or tired or any one of a hundred emotional reasons, none of which has anything to do with physical hunger. If you eat based on emotional hunger, your body will never feel satisfied by food. This is why many people think that they never feel full – they never get the signal to stop eating because they were hungry for emotional fulfilment.

An emotion is a bit like someone knocking on your door to deliver a message. If the message is urgent it knocks loudly; if it's very urgent it knocks very loudly; if it is very urgent and you don't answer the door, it knocks louder and louder and louder until you open the door or it breaks it down. Either way, the emotion will continue to come up until it's done its job. As soon as you 'open the door' by listening to the emotional message and taking appropriate action, the emotion will simply go away.

The good news is that with this new understanding, you don't have to be a victim any more. In future if you are tempted to go and eat a snack, stop and ask yourself this question:

Am I really hungry or do I just want to change the way I feel?

If it turns out that what you actually want is a change in the way that you feel, no amount of food will work as well as applying the simple techniques in this book and on the mind-programming CD.

One additional thought
I am continually surprised at the number of women (and occasionally men) I work with who realize that their initial weight gain coincided with a traumatic incident from the past, ranging from episodes of sexual abuse to seemingly innocuous teasing leading to embarrassment in front of their peers.

While the techniques in this book and on the mind-programming CD will help, they are not intended as a substitute for professional guidance. If you suspect this could apply to you, speak to your doctor and ask them to recommend an appropriate therapist.

Pattern Three: Faulty Programming

If you are overweight it's not your fault – it's the natural result of your current mental programming, and no diet, pill, shake or 'how-to' book can change that. The only way to lose weight and keep it off is to go to the unconscious mind and change your relationship with food for ever.

So relax. You are not crazy, you are not broken, and you

'I got fed up waking up every morning obsessing about food. Since I started using Paul's system I don't. It's great!'

JANET COBB,
TRAINER

are not a bad person. You have simply developed some very unproductive habits. The good news is that once you learn to re-programme your mind, it will be just as simple to develop new habits of thinking and acting that will guarantee your success.

You don't even have to believe that it will work. Just follow my instructions and you will not only lose weight but stop obsessing about food for ever.

In just a few minutes, I'm going to share with you the four most important things you will ever learn about losing weight and keeping it off for life. But before we get started I want you to stop for a moment and do the following thought experiment:

THE POWER OF PERSPECTIVE

Go to near the end of your life. Imagine that it is many years from now and you decided NOT to follow my instructions and begin losing weight. Instead, you carried on trying one diet after another, continuing to gain weight and lose your precious vitality year after year after year ...

- What were the consequences of that decision on your health?

Cont ...

- What were the consequences on your relationships?
- What were the consequences on your sense of well-being?
- How do you feel in your body?

Now . . . Take a few moments to imagine following this programme and easily reaching and maintaining your target weight.

- How good does this feel?
- How much energy do you have?
- What are you able to do?
- What clothes are you able to wear?
- Who are you with? What are you doing? (Besides that . . .)
- Exactly what will it be like when you have lived at your target weight for years and years?

Now . . . STOP!

It's time to decide. If you want to hang on to your excuses and your excess weight, you may as well put the book down now.

But if you're ready finally to get that monkey off your back (and those inches off your waist), know that what you do from this moment onwards is entirely up to you. So let's get started!

Kate Howlett
LOST 4½ STONE

BEFORE   **AFTER**

Before I started doing the Paul McKenna weight-loss system I tried every sort of diet - fat counting, calorie counting, I even tried not eating until after five o'clock at night. I had reached a point where I had given up, I was fat. It ran in my family. What could I do about it? Then a colleague said to me that she had done the Paul McKenna system and that she was feeling really good, so I thought I would give it a try. What did I have to lose?

Once I started doing it I was amazed how easy it was to lose weight and I soon realized that it was not a diet, just a different way of looking at food. I now really enjoy my food, rather than spending all my time thinking about it and then wolfing it down, as I used to do. I now eat when I'm hungry and I get much more out of the whole eating experience. The only problem is that when I am in restaurants I often find that the portions are too big and I have to explain that the food was good, but that I couldn't eat it all because I felt full.

I find that I have much more energy now, partly, I'm sure, because I'm no longer carrying the extra weight round with me, but mainly because when I listen to the CD it says that I'll have more energy when I wake up and I do. I now enjoy walking my son to school. I always used to take the car. One of my greatest pleasures is shopping for clothes. I always used to walk round the shops feeling depressed because I knew that if they had my size I would look awful, but now I really enjoy looking at the clothes because I know that they'll look good on me.

Since doing the Paul McKenna weight-loss system I feel much more positive about life and everything that I approach. The weight loss is like an added bonus to the way the whole system makes me feel.

Kate Howlett

•

CHAPTER TWO

The Simplest Weight-Loss System in the World™

Learning to trust your body

Your body is smarter than any diet on earth, but with volumes of information all around us about how the 'wrong' foods will adversely affect our health or make us put on weight, it can be difficult to see, hear or feel what your body is telling you. In addition, many of us have been so conditioned to think of our bodies as bad or wrong that learning to trust your body can seem a monumental task.

In fact, nothing could be further from the truth. It's not that anything new can't seem a bit difficult at first. Every new activity works this way, from learning to tie your shoelaces to learning to drive a car. In the beginning, you need to consciously learn and apply each step. Then it begins to get easier and easier, and before you know it, you can just do it without even having to think about it.

> 'It definitely works! I am amazed how quickly and easily the weight has come off.'
>
> ANN CARR,
> COMMUNICATIONS
> OFFICER

Putting the force of habit to work for you

When it comes to losing weight and keeping it off, habit is most people's worst enemy. For you, it will be different. We're going to re-condition your habits and make them work for you. What I am about to explain to you is all you really need to change the way you eat for ever. The mind-programming techniques throughout this book and on the CD will reinforce those new habits as the changes begin happening almost immediately.

As you follow the instructions I am about to give you, it will become easier to make smart choices about what and how much to eat in any situation. Soon, you will find yourself eating this way automatically.

How to eat like a naturally thin person

One of the most interesting things I discovered in my research with naturally thin people is how seldom they thought about food. With the exception of imagining what they would most enjoy eating when they were actually hungry, it rarely came up. As a matter of fact, the most striking thing I discovered is how simple making good food choices is for them. Essentially, there are four 'golden rules' they all seemed to follow intuitively. And now they're yours – four simple guiding principles that will help you to make the right food choices in every situation for the rest of your life.

GOLDEN RULE NUMBER 1

When you are hungry, EAT

Why would anyone eat if they weren't hungry?

Well, you may have already guessed that one of the main reasons people eat when they do is simply habit. Like all your other faulty programming, the habit of eating only at prescribed times throughout the day is one of the main culprits in ignoring and overriding your body's innate wisdom.

In fact, many people are so desensitized to their body's messages that they've forgotten how to pay attention. If you read the title of this section and said to yourself 'but I'm hungry all the time!' or 'but I'm never hungry!' this may be what has happened to you. Fortunately, as soon as you begin to make friends with your body again, you will once again be able to recognize the subtle and not so subtle signs of authentic hunger.

How starving yourself can actually make you fat

Ever wondered what's inside a camel's hump? It's fat – stored fat. Camels store fat because they don't know how long they're going to go between meals. When you starve yourself by not eating when you're hungry, your body does the same thing. In fact, if you've been trying to lose weight for a while, your body is probably stuck in continual fat-storage mode.

Similarly, when you starve your body it goes into survival mode because it thinks there is a famine and stores fat in your cells, 'just in case'. Over time, your body begins to leach more fat from whatever foods you do eat. There may be only a few grams of fat in that 'Weight Watchers' lasagne, but if you're eating at 'mealtimes' instead of when you're hungry, your body will do whatever it takes to grab on to that fat and put it where it can store it until later – generally your stomach if you're a man and your hips and thighs if you're a woman.

> 'It was shocking that 7 pounds dropped off within a week and stayed off.'
>
> FIONA ELLIOTT, IT CONSULTANT

That's partly why thin people can eat a lot and not put on weight – they aren't starving themselves so their bodies can either make use of or easily eliminate excess fat from their food.

In addition, consistently overriding your body's natural call for food alters your metabolism. A faster metabolism burns more calories throughout the day, but when you stop yourself from eating when you're hungry, your metabolism slows down so your body can conserve energy. This leads to feelings of lethargy, which many people experience as a mild depression.

If all that wasn't enough, not eating when you're hungry sets up dysfunctional patterns of thinking in the unconscious mind in relation to food. This subtle tension around food sets up a powerful neuro-chemical change in the brain that leads to false hunger signals and patterns of craving and bingeing. The vicious cycle is in motion – the less you trust your body, the less trustworthy your body's messages become.

There is, however, some very good news:

All you need to do to reset your body's innate wisdom is to eat whenever you feel hungry.

Within a few days, your metabolism will stabilize and your body will relax, taking only those nutrients it truly needs to meet the requirements of the moment and easily eliminating the rest.

GOLDEN RULE NUMBER TWO

EAT WHAT YOU WANT, not what you think you should

In a fascinating experiment performed in the 1930s, scientists gave a group of toddlers unlimited twenty-four/seven access to a vast range of foods from ice cream to spinach, essentially allowing them to create their own diet over a period of thirty days based on their own sense of what they wanted to eat and when.

The result?

While they each chose different foods at different times, every single child in the study wound up eating what was considered to be a balanced diet over the course of the month.

Similarly, many women have had the experience of unusual food cravings during pregnancy. The reason a pregnant woman will crave everything from ice cream to pickled onions is that her body is telling her exactly what it needs from moment to moment to 'build a baby'.

Resistance is futile

As soon as you tell yourself not to eat certain foods (usually because you've been told they're bad for you), you upset the natural balance of your relationship to them. Rather than wanting it less, that 'forbidden food' instantly becomes more attractive to you. The inner battle between your positive intention and your resistance to being controlled (even by yourself) can be exhausting. As you begin to make peace with food and learn to listen to the wisdom of your body, you experience freedom from the tension and guilt that comes from NOT following your intuition.

Also, as you stop resisting and start to follow your natural intuitions about what to eat when, you may notice your tastes changing.

'Paul's system has completely changed my life. I no longer constantly think of food. I am thrilled!'

ALEXANDRA SIMMONS, PA

For example, many people fear that if they allow themselves to eat whatever they want when they want, they'll wind up living on a diet of chocolate, pizza and cake. However, studies and my own experience of working with thousands of successful weight losers have demonstrated that when you practise eating what you want over time, you'll wind up eating a fairly balanced diet.

This is sometimes referred to as the 90/10 balance – 90 per cent of your food will be light and nutritionally sound, and 10 per cent will be 'fun food'. You may even find yourself naturally attracted to the very foods you're 'supposed' to be eating now.

GOLDEN RULE
NUMBER THREE

Eat CONSCIOUSLY and enjoy every mouthful

I've noticed a funny thing about people who are over-weight. They spend all their time thinking about food – except when they're actually eating it. Then they go into a kind of 'eating trance', where they shovel as much food into their mouths as they can without actually chewing or tasting anything.

Strange as it may seem, there is a very good reason for that. Whenever we do something that is essential for our survival, like eating, breathing deeply or making love, we release a 'happy chemical' in our brains called serotonin.

People who are overweight often shovel food into their mouths as quickly as possible in order to get a sero-tonin high. Unfortunately, because they are eating unconsciously, they never notice the signal from their stomach that lets them know that they are full. So they keep on stuffing their faces, expanding their stomachs and putting on weight.

The problem is that even though they feel temporarily high from cramming in lots of food, they feel fat and guilty afterwards. In fact, they feel so bad that they repeat the whole ritual of unconsciously stuffing themselves again in order to anaesthetize the bad feelings they just created!

One of the unique features on my weight-loss pro-gramme is this:

You can eat whatever you want, whenever you want, so long as you fully enjoy every single mouthful.

I cannot emphasize this enough. I mean *really* enjoy it –
savour the taste, and enjoy the wonderful textures and
sensations as you thoroughly chew each mouthful.

Of course, in order to fully enjoy your food you have
to notice that you're eating it. A recent study conducted in
Switzerland showed that when people were blindfolded,
they ate 25 per cent less than when they could see – in
other words, when they weren't looking at the food but
were instead totally concentrating on the taste and texture,
they actually ate less.

This corresponds with what I've noticed on my
weight-loss seminars. After lunch, people will often report
that their food tasted amazing, because for the first time in
ages they were eating slowly and consciously enough to
actually taste it and notice the feeling of being full.

Resetting your thermostat

Here is one simple thing you can do to help yourself
remember to enjoy every mouthful of food:

*For the next two weeks, slow your eating speed
down to about a quarter of what it used to be and
chew each mouthful thoroughly.*

As a child, I remember seeing an advertisement for a
special 'diet fork', which had two lights on it – one red,

one green. The instructions were simple: when the light was green, you could eat; when it was red, you had to put down your fork and wait.

While most of us wouldn't want our eating habits to be at the mercy of a fork, the principle is sound. It's very important to put your knife and fork down between every mouthful, so you can give your body time to notice what it's doing. Of course, if you're not using cutlery, prise your fingers off your sandwich and put it down between each mouthful. When your mouth is empty, you can pick up where you left off.

In this way, you make every bite a conscious choice, instead of shovelling in food on automatic.

Do I really have to chew my food?

You can probably think of a time when you were eating popcorn, nuts or crisps while watching a film or a football match. By the time you 'woke up' and came to your senses, the entire bowl, bag or packet was gone. Making the decision to chew each mouthful makes binge eating nearly impossible, as well as bringing some surprising health benefits.

In the nineteenth century, doctors recommended people chew each mouthful at least twenty times for optimal digestion. Now, modern science has demonstrated why chewing your food is so much healthier. The enzymes in your saliva are actually more intense than those in your stomach, enabling you to break down the larger chunks of food more easily. Not only will your digestion improve and your energy levels pick up, you'll naturally wind up eating less and feeling better.

GOLDEN RULE NUMBER FOUR

When you think you are full, STOP eating

I remember as a kid using my mother's kettle to steam open an envelope. In order to keep the steam rising, I had to hold the 'on' switch down long after the kettle had boiled. Of course, kettles aren't designed to be used that way, and soon the metal thermostat inside the kettle became bent and stopped working properly.

> 'Through Paul's system I have gained more insight. It's not what I eat, but how I eat!'
>
> ANNIE ELLIOT, GP

Fortunately, it was quite easy to fix. All I had to do was go inside and bend the thermostat back into place. Immediately, the kettle began working perfectly again.

The natural design of the human body is to eat when we're hungry and stop when we're satisfied, but many of us are conditioned to eat until we think we're full – or even worse, until whatever food we put on our plate is gone.

To lose weight effortlessly and keep it off, you must begin working with your body and not against it. To get slim and stay slim we need to re-sensitize ourselves to our 'inner thermostat' so we can stop eating when we are full and feel good for the rest of the day.

In reality, when you've eaten enough, your stomach sends a signal – a sensation that says, 'I'm satisfied – that's enough.' Most people experience this gentle, clear, satisfied sensation in their solar plexus (the area below your ribcage but above your stomach).

Of course, if you miss this warm feeling of satisfaction when it first occurs, you'll notice that each subsequent bite of food becomes a little less enjoyable than the one before. The more you pay attention to it, the more obvious it becomes.

Since continuing to eat after this satisfied feeling begins to emanate from your solar plexus produces distinct and ever increasing sensations of discomfort, it is important that as soon as you begin to notice this discomfort, you stop eating immediately, no matter how much or how little food is left on your plate.

When I teach this on my seminars, there is invariably one person who starts to panic and say, 'But what if I'm hungry again ten minutes later?'

The answer is very simple; if you're hungry, EAT. However, you must *eat what you actually want*, not what you think you should; eat CONSCIOUSLY and enjoy every mouthful, and then once again when you even suspect you are full, STOP.

The Hunger Scale

At this point I want to introduce you to an amazing tool that you can use to know exactly when to start eating and when to stop. I call it the hunger scale. The hunger scale goes from one, which is physically faint with hunger, to ten, which is stuffed to the point of nausea.

THE HUNGER SCALE

1 – Physically faint

2 – Ravenous

3 – Fairly hungry

4 – Slightly hungry

5 – Neutral

6 – Pleasantly satisfied

7 – Full

8 – Stuffed

9 – Bloated

10 – Nauseous

Take a few moments right now to look at the hunger scale and tune in to your body. How hungry are you right now?

Each person is different, but as a general rule, you want to eat whenever you notice yourself between 3 and 4 on the scale – that is, when you are fairly hungry, but before you become ravenous. If you wait until you get down to 1 or 2 your body will go into starvation mode and you'll probably wind up eating more than your body needs and storing the excess as fat.

Ideally, you'll want to stop eating at around 6 or 7 on the hunger scale – when you are feeling pleasantly satisfied or full but not yet stuffed or bloated.

Of course, if you have been a serial dieter you may be so used to overriding your body's signals that you may at times 'forget to eat' until you're ravenous or keep eating until you're full or even stuffed before noticing it's time to stop. If you think this might be you, practise tuning in to your body once an hour until you begin to notice differences between different points on the scale.

The more you practise tuning in to your own hunger, the sooner you'll be able to recognize your body's subtle signals long before your stomach growls and your brain starts to get fuzzy.

Changing the habits of a lifetime

I was with a friend of mine recently who had been a serial dieter but only seemed to be getting a little bit fatter and a lot more frustrated each year. In less than six months, he has lost four stone using this system.

At first he wasn't sure if it was working, but he stuck to it and after a couple of weeks he noticed his clothes felt looser. He hadn't even done any of the mind-programming techniques – I had simply taught him the four golden rules that I have just taught you and he started using them.

When we were at dinner recently he only ate about half of his meal – a delicious-looking plate of pasta in a rich, creamy sauce. When I asked him if there was anything wrong with his food, he replied, 'No – it's delicious. But ever since you taught me that bloody system, I can't seem to overeat any more.'

This brings us to another reason why people habitually eat more than their bodies want and need . . .

Resigning from the 'Clean Plate Club'

There are lots of people who are members of what I call the 'clean plate club'. Unless they finish everything put in front of them they believe that they are somehow 'bad'. Eating everything on your plate whether you're still hungry and enjoying it or not is basically giving permission for your weight to be controlled by some kid who's being paid £4 an hour at McDonald's. Let's face it, you wouldn't let a shop assistant tell you how much to spend on clothes, would you?

Like most kids, I was told by my parents to eat everything on my plate because 'there are starving children in India'. Don't underestimate the subtle power of this guilt trip, especially if it was installed at a formative age. Eventually, of course, I realized that it was a con. I used to say, 'How does me being overweight help the starving children? Shall I take a picture of myself fat and send it to them with a note saying, "At least you know the food isn't going to waste?"'

Let me put this one to rest once and for all – contrary to popular parental opinion, eating everything on your plate has been shown to do nothing to contribute to the well-being of starving children in Africa, India or China. If you really want to play your part in putting an end to world hunger, learn to manage your eating so that you eat when you're hungry, enjoy every mouthful, and stop when you think you're full. You'll wind up eating so much less that there'll be more for everyone else.

One of the simplest ways to give up your membership of the clean plate club for good is simply to deliberately leave a bit of food on your plate, even if it's just one little chip. In this way, you are sending a new message to your unconscious mind, letting it know for sure that you are changing. Once you've broken the spell (by leaving a little food on your plate each time you eat), you'll feel comfortable eating only until you feel full, even if it means leaving half the food on your plate or more. You'll have less food in your stomach and more control in your life.

(And if you get hungry again later, not to worry – get another plate and leave some food on that one as well!)

The Magic Weight-loss Elixir

There is one other thing that will support you in your efforts to eat only when you are hungry and stop as soon as you even suspect you are full. Our bodies are made up of roughly 75 per cent water, and that percentage increases to nearly 85 per cent in the all-important area of brain tissue. When the inner mechanism in our body that regulates water levels senses any sort of a current or impending shortage, your body goes into selective water rationing mode. The brain gets first call on the water supply, with each internal organ receiving just enough water to maintain basic functioning.

According to Dr F. Batmanghelidj, author of the ground-breaking work *Your Body's Many Cries for Water*, many of the aches and pains that people experience on a daily basis, including hunger, are actually the preliminary effects of dehydration. This is one of the reasons why sometimes no matter what you eat, it doesn't feel as though it 'hits the spot'.

Because it's virtually impossible to tell the difference between this 'thirst signal' and authentic hunger, it's a good idea to make your first response to hunger pangs a fresh glass of water. If you're not hungry afterwards, it was thirst; if you still are, dig in!

What to expect in the next two weeks

1. It will feel weird

Some people tell me that at first they felt a little bit self-conscious eating slowly and consciously chewing each mouthful, as though other people were staring at them. As the saying goes, 'you would worry less about what other people thought of you if you knew how seldom they did'. Most people are so caught up in their own heads they don't even notice what's going into their mouths, let alone what's going on with yours.

Also, people who know you as a serial dieter may notice the pizza, bacon, and chocolate on your plate and smirk, thinking that you've 'fallen off another diet'.

This time, the last laugh will be on them. As it becomes easier and easier to eat consciously, your food will taste better and better and you will enjoy the wonderful feeling of satisfaction that comes from being in control of your eating.

In a society as filled with mixed messages about eating and body image as ours, what is considered 'normal' may be a long way from what is actually natural. While it may feel a bit odd at first to re-programme your body to eat in a new, more intuitive way, it is important to recognize you are actually moving towards a more natural way of eating.

This is why it is sustainable – unlike diets, which go against your natural urge to eat when you are hungry and stop when you are full, the simplest weight-loss system in the world works *with* your body.

2. You will feel good

One of the most consistent benefits people report from using the simplest weight-loss system in the world is that they feel better – better in their bodies and better in themselves.

Here's what to expect:

- For the first time in ages you will feel more in control around food.
- The pressure of worrying about what to eat and when will be gone. It will be liberating to know you are free from the slavery of obsessing about food.
- You will see that it truly is possible for you to lose weight easily.
- You will realize that slim people are not different to you. We are all the same in our ability to lose weight.

In fact you will be amazed at how easy it is!

Because you are not spending so much energy worrying about food you will have more energy available for your life. This extra energy is one of the signs that the system is working perfectly.

3. You will wonder how well it's working

People who have successfully used this system often say that within the first couple of weeks they weren't sure if it was working. Whether you feel like you are eating more than before, or that you're not eating nutritionally balanced meals, or even like nothing much is different. . .

> *Relax! As long as you are following the four golden rules, it's working.*

It's normal to have doubts simply because you are doing something very different from what you have done before. Soon, as you begin to notice increased levels of energy, a slight change in how your clothes fit, and a general sense of well-being in your body, you will realize that everything is working perfectly. Remember, you have already tried all sorts of other systems, diets or techniques and they haven't worked, or they've only worked for a short time. By committing to my system for the next two weeks, you've got nothing to lose except weight.

4. You will at some point forget to follow my instructions and break at least one if not all four of the golden rules

It's important for you to know that YOU WILL have a slip or two along the way, shoving in a sandwich on the run, gorging yourself on chocolate digestives, eating to calm your nerves or even a full-on binge.

At this point you have a choice:

You can beat yourself up (like you've done in the past) and give up, telling yourself that you're a worthless piece of shit and you're never going to change.

Or

You can RELAX, smile, remind yourself that I told you this would happen, and return to eating what you want when you are hungry, consciously enjoying each mouthful, and stopping when you think you are full. No matter what happens, always go back to following my instructions.

Weighing yourself

Let me offer you one final note of caution. Over the years that I have been working with weight-loss clients, I have noticed how many people are absolutely obsessed with weighing themselves. Some do it every day; some even do it after every meal, treating the scales like the lottery, expecting to see that suddenly they have lost a couple of stone since lunchtime.

> *You cannot get an accurate reading on your weight loss by checking every day.*

Each time you climb on to those scales, all you are doing is setting yourself up to feel bad. Everybody's weight goes up and down all the time – even slim people. In fact, naturally thin people rarely if ever weigh themselves. Most of them couldn't tell you what they weigh if you paid them.

Because weight can fluctuate as much as ten pounds up or down from environmental factors, water retention and even atmospheric pressure, it is actually the least reliable measure on the road to becoming thin. So it is important that you DO NOT WEIGH YOURSELF for the next two weeks.

I actually recommend that you give up the scales for life – you'll know you're thin because you look great and you feel wonderful. However, if you absolutely must weigh yourself, leave at least TWO weeks between each weighing.

When an aeroplane flies from one place to another it doesn't fly in a straight line – it's always adjusting its course. Despite the fact that it's off course as much as 91 per cent of the time, it always knows where it's going.

It's the same with losing weight – while some days will be better than others and sometimes you will feel more confident about your weight than others, if you keep your eye on the prize and keep following the guidelines, YOU WILL LOSE WEIGHT and keep it off, for as long as you use this system.

Can it really be this simple?

Yes! Let's review the four elements of the system:

1. Eat whenever you are hungry
2. Eat only what you want, never what you think you 'should'
3. Eat consciously and enjoy every mouthful
4. Stop when you even think your body is full

That is all you need to do in order to lose weight and keep it off for life. And if you're truly ready to be thin, I can make it even simpler for you. If you change only one thing about the way that you eat, do this:

Consciously Enjoy Every Mouthful.

By focusing on this one element of the system, everything else will fall into place, because:

- You can't and won't get the full enjoyment out of your food if you're not properly hungry
- You can only truly enjoy your food when you choose only foods you truly enjoy
- Your food will stop being enjoyable if you don't stop eating when your body is full

Maureen Edwards
LOST 18 STONE

BEFORE   **AFTER**

I went to a barbecue one day. It was packed out with people. I'd got up to get some food and I'd piled up my plate (I don't mind admitting now that I had a food addiction – I knew how big I was but I was just addicted to food). Anyway, I'd sat back down and when I needed to get up again I couldn't get out of the chair.

I found out later that when we'd arrived my sister had found me the biggest chair there – it was one of those white plastic outdoor chairs – but I just couldn't get out. I could feel it buckling underneath me and the legs splaying out under my weight, so I shouted for my husband to come and help.

Everyone was laughing and I tried to laugh along too, but the humiliation was breaking my heart. The arms of the chair were embedded in my thighs (72-inch thighs!) and drawing blood. There was blood all over my white trouser suit and in the end I couldn't pretend to laugh any more and I was sobbing my heart out.

It took my husband and another friend to finally get me out, shattering the arm of the chair in the process. It was on the way home in the car, still sobbing, that I decided to do something, and I thought about Paul McKenna's weight-loss CDs because a friend had recommended them.

I wasn't convinced, though, because I'd tried so many diets in the past, and although you always have a little ray of hope that this one will work for you, it usually doesn't.

Anyway, the next morning, still not convinced, I put on a pair of tracky bottoms and a baggy T-shirt, but covered them up with a big coat and went out with a carrier bag so my neighbours would think I was going shopping! I was going on a 2-mile walk, but at the top of the hill I had to phone Ron to come and get me. I was too exhausted to get home and I knew I was too overweight to do it without help. That really was it.

The next day I got hold of Paul McKenna's CDs, went upstairs to play them, and I can honestly say that's the day my life changed.

Now I take him to bed every night! I'm the manager of a gym and some days I take up to three aerobics classes a day. I'm so full of life now. Sometimes I think back to not even being able to reach round to wipe my own backside! I know that sounds disgusting but that's how big I was! I've gone from 28 stone to 10 stone in two years and every day I still feel great about how different life feels. And I help other people too. I'm the Mo in Motivation! And if I can do it, anybody can.

Maureen Edwards

CHAPTER THREE

•

Programme Your Mind to Slim Your Body

Changing the habits of a lifetime

I know there have been many times in the past when you've done your best to eat sensibly, but no matter how hard you tried, you couldn't stick with it. And you probably thought that in some way it was your fault – if only you had more will-power, you wouldn't be overweight.

Based on the latest scientific data, I can address that issue once and for all:

Rubbish!

The truth is that it's nearly impossible to break a habit with will-power alone – you have to re-programme your mind. With the right programmes in place, doing the right thing is easy; with the wrong programmes running your mind, it's virtually impossible.

Over the years, I have helped people change life-long compulsions in a matter of minutes and proved that even the most die-hard addiction will succumb to effective re-programming. Yet until you've experienced it for yourself, this may seem a bit different. After all, if lasting changes can happen this quickly and this easily, why haven't you been able to do it in the past?

It all boils down to a simple psychological rule:

Your imagination is far more powerful than your will.

To give yourself a quick experience of this, imagine a piece of chocolate cake (or your favourite food) in front of you. Next, tell yourself with all your will-power that you are not going to eat it. Then imagine the taste of that chocolatey icing as it melts on your tongue. Can you feel your will weakening yet?

Next, once again imagine that piece of chocolate cake (or your favourite food) in front of you. Now, imagine the cake is covered in maggots – slimy, wriggling maggots. Notice the foul smell emanating from the maggots (or is it the cake?). Has the cake lost some of its appeal?

That's the power of your imagination in action. In fact, it's through your imagination that you actually make all your best decisions about what you are going to eat. When you read the menu in a restaurant, you mentally taste all the food in your mind before you decide what to have. That's why restaurants go to such trouble to describe their food in appetizing terms. For example, which would you rather have for dinner this evening: 'Goujons of sole lightly sautéed and served in a delicate lemon sauce' or 'dead fish'?

The focus factor

Take a moment now to ask yourself:

What do I want in relation to my body?

If you're like most people, you answered something like 'to lose weight' or 'to get rid of my love handles' or 'to not be so fat'.

One of the most basic psychological rules in life is, 'You always get more of what you focus on.' Yet in each one of the examples above, your mind has to focus on what you *don't* want in order to make sense of it – the weight you want to lose, the 'love handles' that you secretly hate, or the fat you want to leave behind. This not only reinforces the image people have of themselves as fat, it tends to leave them feeling helpless, hopeless and unmotivated.

When you redirect your focus exclusively on to what you want – a slim, fit, healthy body – you are sending a message to your unconscious mind to find and explore every possible opportunity to move towards your goal. By clarifying and vividly imagining exactly what it is you want for yourself, you are beginning the process of training your mind and body to give it to you.

Now, the more specific you are, the better this works. If you just say, *I'd like to be thinner*, your mind might interpret that as meaning you want to lose one pound. So describe exactly what it is that you want . . .

For example:

I want to lose four stone in the next four months.

Or,

I want to feel comfortable in a size-eight dress.

Or my personal favourite,

I want to look great naked!

Self-image and the self-fulfilling prophecy

Remember, all you need to do to reach your goal is:

1. Eat when you're hungry
2. Eat what you actually want
3. Eat consciously and enjoy each mouthful
4. Stop when you think you're full

So why keep reading?

Because the techniques that follow will make the whole process happen even more easily and allow you to feel significantly better about yourself as well. In other words:

> *We are not only what we eat,*
> *but what we think as well.*

In the 1960s the famous plastic surgeon Maxwell Maltz found that after many of his operations, the self-esteem and confidence levels of his patients rose dramatically. However, for a few people the operations didn't seem to make any difference. After a great deal of exploration, Dr Maltz concluded that those patients who didn't experience a change in their levels of well-being were 'scarred on the inside'. They saw themselves as unworthy, bad or hopeless, and the fact that their appearance had changed on the outside made no difference to the image they held of themselves on the inside. They had what he called 'an impoverished self-image'.

Your self-image is how you see yourself in your imagination. It's the blueprint that determines everything about you, from how motivated, intelligent and confident you are willing to let yourself be to how much weight you are willing to carry around with you or lose.

The reason our self-image has such a powerful influence on our behaviour is that it is self-reinforcing. For example, we've all met people who are not classically good-looking but have an aura of attractiveness. Because they think of themselves as attractive they carry themselves well, dress to bring out their most attractive features, and have the confidence to speak to anyone. This self-confidence makes them attractive to others, who respond positively to them, which reinforces their image of themselves as attractive.

Equally, there are plenty of people who think of themselves as unattractive, and unconsciously sabotage any attempts to appear attractive. After all, if you truly believe you are unattractive, why take the time to dress mutton up as lamb? However, if you don't do what it takes to represent yourself at your best, people will inevitably find you unattractive.

Either way, your self-image has worked perfectly, 'proving' itself right by guiding you to act consistently with who you believe yourself to be.

Nearly every overweight person has a self-image that says they will always be fat. While they may say they would prefer to be thin, they often think that thin people are somehow different from them, and the goal seems almost unattainable.

How do you change the pattern?

By getting into the habit of focusing your attention on what you actually DO want. Like it or not, you're going to need to get used to thinking of yourself with an attractive body!

See yourself slim

Recent scientific research in the United States and Europe has conclusively shown that visualization techniques dramatically enhance your ability to lose weight. As you vividly imagine yourself slim and rehearse your path to your ideal weight, you send a message to your brain that affects your energy levels, your motivation and your metabolism. Those changes cause physical sensations, which in turn affect your thoughts and emotions, which in turn reinforce the programming you are giving your brain. It's a positive feedback system, and every element of the system gets to feel good as you lose weight.

As I guide you through these next two exercises, I am going to be instructing you to visualize. This is something everyone already has the ability to do. To prove this to yourself answer the following questions:

1. What does your front door look like?

2. What colour is it?

3. Which side is the handle on?

In order to answer any of these questions, you had to visualize – to go into your imagination and make pictures. Now, for 99 per cent of people, these mental images will not be as real as reality – and that's a good thing. People who can't tell the difference between the pictures in their head and what they see in the world are in trouble.

Your perfect body

Here's a simple but powerful exercise that will train your unconscious mind to help you lose weight and keep it off. Before you do this exercise read through all the steps first.

1. Stop for a moment and imagine you are watching a movie of a thin, happy, confident you.

2. Watch that thinner you doing the things that you do in your daily life and accomplishing them with ease. Imagine this new you eating just the right amount, moving their body regularly, and handling their emotional needs quickly and easily.

Cont ...

- How does that other you talk to themselves?

- What kind of voice tone do they use?

- How do they carry themselfes?

- How do they move?

3. If the movie is not yet exactly how you want things to be, make the adjustments that make you feel great. Allow your intuition to be your guide.

4. When you are satisfied with the other you, step into it. Take the new perspective and behaviours into you.

5. Now run the movie and imagine being in all of your daily situations and view them from your new perspective. Think through what it's like to have this new perspective and what it will help you to achieve. How are things going to be so much better now?

Repetition, repetition, repetition

Remember, repetition is the key to success. When we repeat an action, a neural pathway is created in the brain and each repetition reinforces it. As you think of yourself as slim and healthy you are sending signals to your unconscious mind to behave, to feel and to eat like a slim person. As your body gets lighter you will feel more sensitive, more energetic and more alive.

Do this exercise every morning and before long, it will become a healthy habit. The more you do this the sooner you will start to feel better and change the way you feel about yourself for the better. Each time you do it, you will be one step closer to your ideal weight.

This exercise focuses your mind on your target, making it more powerful and more and more compelling, so that every time you say no to the foods you no longer wish to eat and yes to those foods you actually want, you will feel more of this delightful lightness and know you are one step closer to your ideal weight.

In addition, each time you listen to the special mind-programming CD, you will be reinforcing all the gains you make each time you take the time to see yourself slim.

Claire Singh
LOST 6½ STONE

BEFORE **AFTER**

My weight has been a problem for most of my adult life, and in the past I have tried every single diet hundreds of times. Around Christmas last year I was at my lowest ebb, and I could see no way out of the vicious circle of eating and gaining weight, and generally my poor relationship with food. If you had asked me what I ate in a day, I would have been honest and told you, but I can guarantee that I would not have included everything, because I ate without thinking. I simply did not register it all. I would eat whether I was hungry or not, and didn't even think about it. It was a slippery slope to nowhere.

My mum paid for Paul's workshop as a Christmas present, and I thought I would go as I had nothing to lose. I will never forget that day. Sitting on the tube on the way home, I felt so inspired. It was simple, yet such a huge revelation, as if someone had just woken me up and said, 'Here are the answers.' It seemed so obvious: 'Just follow these simple steps and off you go ...' For the first time in my life I actually thought about the food I ate, before and while eating it!

At the same time as beginning my new way of life, I started going to the gym, where I was helped by Mike, my personal trainer. The exercise seemed like a natural accompaniment to my new 'normal' lifestyle, and I was weighed regularly, which was also a great incentive and motivator.

It took a bit of time to believe that I could do this – it seemed so simple, and I needed to realize that it was not a dream. But my life has changed so much, it's incredible. I have had so much support from my fantastic mum and my friends. It's just brilliant. I feel that, at twenty-eight, I'm beginning to live the life I should have had. Every single area of my life has changed. I'm confident in every way, and shopping for clothes is now fun, not a nightmare!

I lead a very active life, and I now view food in a completely different way. I know now that food is fuel for the body, not a life crutch. Ever since attending Paul's workshop, I eat a lot less. I actually think about what I eat and become full more easily. I don't eat junk food and have even improved my cooking skills!! Not only do I feel a lot better from losing so much weight, but I'm also more in tune with my body, and I no longer suffer from bad health generally, and a poor digestive system.

I will always be grateful for the life-changing experience, and don't take my 'second chance' for granted. When I'm having a busy time I just listen to Paul's CD. It's useful for refocusing my mind, and it's supportive. This experience really has been life-changing. It's like someone said, 'Here's the key to the rest of your life ...'

Claire Singh

CHAPTER FOUR

•

Overcoming Emotional Eating

Recognizing emotional hunger

As I mentioned in Chapter One, emotional eating is one of the primary causes of obesity in the world. Yet book after book and programme after programme attempt to address the issue by telling you what you should or shouldn't eat. That's like trying to fix a broken leg by telling the person they shouldn't have fallen down! Instead of going outside yourself and asking the so-called diet experts 'what should I eat?' you need to go inside and ask yourself 'what's eating me?'

One of the most common mistakes people make when they first start out on my system is to confuse emotional hunger with physical hunger. This is because until we become more attuned to our bodies, the two feel remarkably similar.

Here are a couple of pointers to help you make a clear distinction every time:

1. Emotional hunger is sudden and urgent; physical hunger is gradual and patient

Have you ever had the experience of having a sudden, desperate craving for food? If you track back in your mind, you'll find that only moments before the 'hunger' arrived, you were having an argument with yourself in your mind. In order to not deal with whatever feelings are going on in your body, people learn to bury those feelings with food.

Physical hunger, on the other hand, is gradual. You may notice a gentle griping in your tummy, or even a deep rumbling. If you continue to ignore your hunger, you'll probably experience light-headedness or even sadness, anger and tiredness. The earlier you learn to pick up on your body's 'hints' that it needs fuel, the easier it will be to separate out these two signals.

2. Emotional hunger cannot be satisfied with food; physical hunger can

In a fascinating study at the University of Hertfordshire, Professor Ben Fletcher achieved spectacular results by teaching people to respond to their 'hunger pangs' by going out and doing something in the world – turning off the TV and going for a walk, speaking with a friend, or even going out to a movie. This fed their emotional hunger, and allowed them to quiet the emotional signals their body was sending them. As those emotional signals quietened, it was easy for people to hear and respond to the physical feelings of hunger and fullness.

If you are eating and eating and never feeling satisfied, it's because you don't need food – you need to change your feelings. When you're hungry for good feelings (or at least a temporary masking of bad feelings), no amount of food will do the trick. This is an additional way in which emotional hunger differs from physical hunger – when you address the root cause of emotional hunger, it doesn't come back again four hours later!

The cause of emotional hunger

Regardless of its specific manifestations, the feelings that underlie emotional hunger invariably come down to one thing, a secret many people carry with them throughout their lives:

Self-loathing – feeling hopeless, helpless, worthless and unloved

As we have already learned, the mind and body are intimately linked. Recent scientific research has shown that our thoughts have a significant effect upon our health and well-being. We can change biological processes in the body through our imagination and we can certainly change our feelings and moods.

Your harshest critic

I am continually amazed at the self-abuse that most people put themselves through at the start of each day. They'll look at themselves in the mirror in the morning, say 'fat face, fat arms, fat thighs, fat arse', and then go about their day wondering why they don't feel good about themselves.

On my weight-loss seminars I do an exercise where I help people stop the self-abuse and start to appreciate themselves. I ask for a volunteer to look into a mirror and share their internal criticism out loud with the group. Once, I was doing this exercise with a lovely looking lady who saw herself in the mirror and immediately blurted out, 'Fat fucking cow.'

Of course everyone burst out laughing because they could so easily identify with her. When I asked her what she would do if someone walked up to her in the street and said that to her, she replied that she would probably hit them. She wouldn't take it from someone else, but she'd readily insult herself every time she looked in the mirror.

Possibly the most famous guideline for effective living in Western civilization is the so-called 'golden rule', which is generally expressed in some version of 'Do unto others as you would have done unto you'. My candidate for a 'platinum rule' is this:

Do unto yourself as you would have others do unto you.

If anyone else insulted us as openly and crudely as we insult ourselves ('I'm such a stupid idiot', 'I'm so useless', 'I'm such a waste of space', 'God, I'm pathetic', etc.) or punished us as unforgivingly as we punish ourselves ('I can't believe I ate dessert – that's it! I'm going to work out until I throw up!'), we would be up in arms, protesting at the injustice and inhumanity of such cruel and unusual treatment.

But when we treat ourselves that way, we put up with it – mostly because nobody ever told us we didn't have to. Until you realize that there are healthy alternatives to motivating yourself to lose weight by beating yourself up for being fat, you will find it virtually impossible to measure up to your own unrealistically high standards. Fortunately, by seeing self-loathing for what it is, you lessen its power over you and make it possible to address it directly instead of attempting to stuff it down with food. As you begin to see yourself as capable, lovable, and intrinsically worthy, you will continue to feel the pangs of emotional hunger.

When you are feeling low, it is commonplace that friends and family can see your strengths and value even when you do not. We can use this fact to begin the process of loving and valuing ourselves. Here's an exercise to help you begin to change the patterns of self-loathing that most of us have been carrying throughout our lives.

SOMEBODY WHO LOVES YOU

Before you do this exercise read through all the steps first.

1. If it's appropriate, close your eyes and think of someone who loves or deeply appreciates you. Remember how they look, and imagine they are standing in front of you now.

2. Gently step out of your body and into the body of the person who loves you. See through their eyes, hear through their ears, and feel the love and good feelings they have as you look at yourself. Really notice in detail what it is that they love and appreciate about you. Recognize and acknowledge those amazing qualities that perhaps you hadn't appreciated about yourself until now.

3. Step back into your own body and take a few moments to enjoy those good feelings of knowing that you are loved and appreciated exactly as you are.

You can keep that inner feeling with you for hours and hours and re-run this exercise whenever you want to boost it. The more you do it, the easier it becomes, and eventually it becomes automatic to love and feel loved.

The natural design of your body

Did you know that less than one per cent of the women in the world even have the genetic potential for what is considered a 'model figure'? Yet when I meet people who consider themselves to be overweight, they spend an inordinate amount of time comparing themselves to air-brushed magazine images of smiling, anorexically thin women and make themselves feel so bad they need to eat something in order to feel better!

Our bodies contain a natural blueprint for optimal health. Human beings are designed to be around five or six feet tall, and that's why we stop growing in our late teens. No one carries on growing to twenty feet – it wouldn't be natural and it wouldn't be healthy. In the same way, we have a natural shape. If we get too much bigger or smaller than that, it's because we have interfered with the natural design of the body.

It is very common for people to tell me that they don't like their bodies and will do whatever they can to try to ignore them. What they don't realize is that it is important to pay attention – if you want to change how you look, you must first make peace with your natural body. In fact, the more you learn to accept your body as it is, the more you'll be amazed at how effortlessly it changes.

Here's the bottom line:

You've got to make friends with the body you have in order to get the body you want.

Of course you may be looking forward to thinner thighs or a flatter tummy, but it is this same body you are already in that is going to be fitter and slimmer, so you may as well begin making peace with it now.

Anorexia, bulimia and body dysmorphia

(While all of the techniques in this book can make a real difference to the way you feel about yourself and the actions you take, if you suspect or have been told that you are suffering from an eating disorder, you should seek help from an appropriate professional.)

Even though anorexics and bulimics are often painfully thin, they tell themselves how overweight they are and say all kinds of abusive things to themselves when they look in the mirror.

Some of them are able to telescope their vision on to some tiny aspect of themselves, focusing all their self-hate on to that one body part. Others are able to completely hallucinate, similar to those fun-house mirrors at the seaside that make you appear much taller or wider than you really are. This distorted self-image, commonly referred to as 'body dysmorphia' keeps people from truly enjoying life or eating enough. At best it has dire health consequences; at worst it can be fatal.

I worked with a lovely-looking lady on TV who couldn't look at herself in the mirror without bursting into tears. She'd tried every kind of therapy and none of it had worked. Using the techniques that I am about to teach you, she overcame this horrible life-long disorder. In less than an hour, she was able to confidently look at herself in the mirror and see herself as beautiful.

During the change process I asked her to remember a time when she had been paid a compliment. Try as she might, she couldn't think of a single one.

Her partner was present and I suggested she think of a time when he'd said something nice to her. 'That'll be the day!' she said. He looked a little hurt and surprised and replied, 'I say nice things to you all the time.'

Before she had a chance to argue, I jumped in and said, 'I believe him!'

Our self-image acts as a filter for what fits with who

we think we are. Because she had such a poor self-image, whenever anybody said anything nice to her she immediately dismissed it because it didn't fit with who she thought she was.

The sweetest moment in this session came at the end. Although she had been with her partner for several years and they had a child together, they had never got married because she couldn't bear the thought of 'all those people looking at her on her wedding day while she was so hideous'.

After we had taken away the self-hate and she filled herself up with love, I asked her how she felt about getting married now. She turned, smiled at her partner, and said, 'Well, someone will have to ask me.' She was finally able to let in all the love that he had been trying to give her for years.

The friendly mirror

Everyone receives compliments and praise from time to time. Sometimes they may seem trivial, like 'Hey, you're looking great' or 'You look sharp today'. At other times they may seem quite significant, like 'You are so sexy', or 'Do you know how much people respect you?'

Sincere, positive perceptions from others, which you might not have been able to see or fully appreciate from the point of view you had at the time, can be valuable in learning to appreciate your own qualities more fully and enhance your self-esteem now.

The next two techniques will not only help you to eliminate emotional hunger, they will also help you feel better and better about yourself every time you look in the mirror. Read through each technique several times until you know the steps and then go and do it.

THE FRIENDLY MIRROR – PART ONE

Before you do this exercise read through all the steps first.

1. Standing in front of a mirror with your eyes closed, recall a specific time when you were paid a compliment by someone you respect or trust. You don't necessarily need to have believed the compliment at the time but you do need to trust the sincerity of the person who said it. Run through the experience all over again.

2. As you recall the compliment, and the sincerity of the person who said it, pay particular attention to your feelings of trust and regard for the other person.

3. When you feel that as strongly as possible, open your eyes, look in the mirror and really see what they saw. Allow yourself to see what someone else has seen and notice how that feels.

4. Finally, imagine taking a picture of yourself just like that. Imagine taking that picture right into your heart. Keep it there so that you can look at it whenever you want to remind yourself how good you can feel.

When you get comfortable with Part One, you can move on to:

THE FRIENDLY MIRROR – PART TWO

Before you do this exercise read through all the steps first.

1. Each day, spend at least one minute looking at your body in the mirror. In an ideal world, you will do this without clothes, but if that doesn't feel right at first, you may wear anything that reveals your basic shape.

2. Notice what thoughts come up, from 'this is stupid' to 'God, I hate my thighs' to 'hmmm . . . not bad – not bad at all!'

3. Send love, approval and positive energy to the person in the mirror. Let them know that you're on their side, and that your love for them is not dependent on the size of their thighs.

Remember to use these techniques every day and don't be too surprised at how quickly you begin to notice the changes. For many people just moving from self-hate to a state of neutral self-acceptance is life-changing. Eventually, you will get all the way to love, and then the changes become even more dramatic.

As you begin actively to meet your own emotional needs, you will find your emotional hunger begins to diminish. As it does, eating only when you are truly hungry for food will become easier and more natural. You will become noticeably more confident and charismatic. Day by day, you'll find yourself naturally doing things that you used to only dream of.

CHAPTER FIVE

•

The Truth About Exercise

The myth of metabolism

Your metabolism is the speed at which your body produces energy. The faster your metabolism, the faster your body does everything, from adjusting your body temperature to growing your fingernails. And more importantly for our purposes, the faster it will burn off any excess fat, regardless of whether that fat comes from a hearty roast beef platter or your hips, thighs and stomach.

> '*I have used Paul's techniques to help me run a five-kilometre race. The weight came off with hardly any effort.*'
>
> KATHY TREVELYAN,
> TOUR GUIDE

The rate at which your metabolism is currently running is called your 'basal metabolic rate', and it is the primary determinant in how many calories your body will burn off throughout the day.

One of the great myths of the weight-loss world is the myth of metabolism, which says:

Certain people will find it more difficult to lose weight than others because of their genetically pre-determined basal metabolic rate.

The way you've probably heard it is more like this:

I can't lose weight because I have a slow metabolism.

However, your metabolism is not fixed – it can and will change throughout your life in response to how you eat and use your body. In this chapter, I will show you not only how to speed up your metabolism but how to 'super-charge' it too, enabling you to increase your basal metabolic rate and burn more fat and calories throughout the day and even while you sleep!

Can't I just change my diet to boost my metabolism?

There are very few 'sure things' in life, but I want to offer you one here:

If you continue to diet, you will gain weight and keep it on for life.

I know this is a controversial thing to say, but as we go a bit deeper into our understanding of metabolism, I think you'll quickly see that you must simply give up.

Remember it works like this: if you starve your body, it goes into self-preservation mode, also known as 'fat storage' mode. Your metabolism will slow right down and you will feel sluggish and completely uninterested in exercise or any other physical activity. This is because when you are starving yourself, your body will try to compensate by shutting down your metabolism. It wants to conserve energy, so it will slow all your energy systems down to a minimum and leach anything it can turn into fat (stored energy) in your body.

On the flip side, when you eat whenever you are hungry, your body learns it has plenty of fuel. It cranks up your metabolism so that energy can be used quickly and efficiently. Because it knows the energy will be replenished as needed, it doesn't bother to store any additional fat reserves, and you not only look thin but are filled with energy as well.

The truth about exercise

The traditional way to increase your basal metabolic rate is through exercise. But before you throw your hands up in horror, realize that 'exercise' is simply this:

Anything you do that causes you to breathe more deeply than you normally would and/or causes your heart rate to speed up.

Can you think of any enjoyable ways to get your heart pumping and breathe more deeply than you are breathing now?

If so, you are already on your way to making supercharging your metabolism an easy and enjoyable part of your life.

When I ask people about exercise they think about running on a track or pumping iron. It always makes me laugh when people tell me on my weight-loss seminars that they never exercise. 'Don't you get out of bed in the morning?' I ask them. 'How about walking around your home? Do you ever leave your flat or house? Does somebody carry you or do you do it on your own two feet?'

The fact is, you already 'exercise' all day every day, simply by moving your body. The key to supercharging your metabolism (and in so doing, speeding up the rate at which your body burns through calories and fat) is simply to move more than you are currently doing.

Simple steps to success

Our bodies are made with muscles that are designed to be used. Because lots of us work at desks and travel by car, bus and train, we don't use our muscles as much as our ancestors used theirs. We have inherited all the healthy genes for fitness and a fast-burning metabolism, but we've fallen out of the habit of using them as much or as often as we could.

In an interesting study, researcher and author Dr James Hill discovered that the average number of steps taken per day by women between the ages of eighteen and fifty was only a little over 5,000. (For men, the average was closer to 6,000 steps a day.) Even more intriguingly, the study revealed that people who were overweight took 1,500 to 2,000 fewer steps a day than those who maintained a healthy weight.

Think about that for a moment – **only 2,000 extra steps a day can make the difference between being over-weight and being slim**! That's about the distance it would take for you to walk four city blocks. The more steps you take, the more calories you use up, and the increased speed of your metabolism from those extra steps will continue to burn away your fat while you rest or sleep.

While some doctors recommend you maintain at least 10,000 steps a day, I have known people to make remarkable strides with their weight loss by increasing their step count to as much as 20,000 a day.

If you'd like to figure out how many steps you already walk each day, you can purchase a simple pedometer (step counter) at almost any sports shop for about one pound. Just attach it to your clothing when you get started in the morning and find out how many steps you currently take in a typical day. Aim to increase the number of steps by 2,000 a week until you hit a comfortably maintainable target.

Is that really it?

The biggest exercise myth in the world is the idea of 'No Pain No Gain'. The reality of exercise is, 'No Effort, No Gain; a little bit of effort, tremendous gain'. But effort should never be confused with pain. Pain is bad, and if you feel any pain at all during exercise, you need to stop immediately. It really is that simple. If you want to exercise regularly, you need to enjoy your moving of your body, both as you're doing it and after.

Now let's take a look at some of the additional benefits of exercise. Studies have shown that regular exercisers not only lose weight, but they feel great. This is because exercise releases one of the best stress-reducing drugs available – your own natural endorphins. Here's how it works . . .

Your body does not distinguish between an emotional threat and a physical one. So even when you're just worrying about bad things happening, your body prepares to protect itself by fighting or running away – but often there is no one to fight and nowhere to run to. The body gets worked up but cannot find a way to release its tension.

Each time you exercise, you are helping your body release the tension of the stress response, making it feel calmer, safer and healthier. In addition, regular exercise triggers the body's natural impulse to rest, relaxation, and recuperation, also known as the *parasympathetic response.*

The parasympathetic response is the sweet, soft feeling you get in your muscles when you have finished some heavy work or vigorous movement. You also feel a natural high caused by the release of endorphins, the body's natural opiates.

That in turn positively affects your mood, making you emotionally clearer and more able to function well – to concentrate, to relax and to sleep soundly.

So any time you're feeling less than your best, you can give yourself an easy, positive boost by simply taking ten to fifteen minutes of brisk exercise – any movement (including walking) that speeds up your heart rate and gets you breathing more deeply than you are breathing right now.

Unleashing the athlete within

Taking exercise helps you to build muscle, lose fat and feel great. It contributes to clearer skin, enhanced mental clarity, better athletic performance and an increased sex drive. Certain hormones released during exercise have been shown to slow and even reverse the ageing process.

So why aren't you already doing more of it?

Well, it's probably because in the past you thought about exercise and imagined yourself huffing and puffing on an exercise machine, listening to a maniacal aerobics instructor shouting 'feel the burn', or looking into a wall-sized mirror surrounded by people who look so much better than you that you just want to go home and throw up.

Simply put, until you deliberately root out your negative associations with exercise and install new positive ones, you will continue to tell yourself you 'should' do it and beat yourself up for not listening.

As I guide you through this next exercise, we are going to make the idea of moving your body much more appealing, using the psychological power of vivid visualization and simple association to create a super-state of motivation to take exercise that you can trigger whenever you want.

You are going to do this by creating a trigger, or anchor, which will put you in touch with feeling great. My personal choice of anchor is squeezing together the thumb and middle finger on one hand. You choose the same anchor, or use a different finger if you like. It's easy and inconspicuous and you can do it anywhere.

Here's how it works . . .

MOTIVATION POWER! – PART ONE

In a moment we are going to remember some times when you felt totally motivated, or anything else that you REALLY enjoy doing. Then we are going to create an association between those feelings and this squeeze of your fingers by repeating them together, over and over again.

Before you do this exercise read through all the steps first.

1. Rate on a scale of 1 to 10 how strong your motivation to exercise is. 1 is the weakest, 10 the strongest.

2. Think of something that you are already motivated to do. It may be something you feel particularly passionate about, like your favourite hobby or pastime, a political cause, being with a loved one or spending time with your family.

   If nothing springs to mind immediately ask yourself, if you had won a lottery jackpot – how motivated would you be to go and collect the cheque? Or how motivated would you be to save the life of your closest friend? Or if the most attractive person in the world asked you out on a date – how motivated would you be to say 'yes'?

Cont ...

3. Whatever motivates you most right now, I'd like you to visualize the scene – seeing it through your own eyes as though it's here now. See again what you would see, hear what you would hear, and feel exactly how being motivated feels.

   Now notice all the details of the scene. Make the colours richer, bolder and brighter. Make the sounds clearer and the feelings stronger. As the feelings build to a peak, squeeze together your finger and thumb.

4. Keep going through that motivational movie. As soon as it finishes, start it again, all the time feeling that motivation and squeezing your thumb and finger together. See what you saw, hear what you heard, and feel that motivation.

5. STOP! Relax your fingers. Move about a bit.

Are you ready to test your motivation trigger? Squeeze your thumb and finger together and relive that good feeling now. It's important to realize it may not feel as intense, but you can increase your feelings of motivation every time you do this exercise.

MOTIVATION POWER! – PART TWO

Before you do this exercise read through all the steps first.

1. It's time to make the association between feeling motivated and moving your body. Squeeze your thumb and finger together and remember what it's like to feel motivated. Now imagine yourself moving your body easily and effortlessly throughout the day. Imagine things going perfectly, going exactly the way you want them to go, finding more and more opportunities to enjoy moving your body in enjoyable ways. See what you'll see, hear what you'll hear, and feel how good it feels. As soon as you have done that go through it again, still squeezing together your finger and thumb, permanently associating motivation to exercise.

2. Finally, on a scale of 1 to 10, how motivated do you feel to move your body? The higher the number, the easier you will find it to incorporate exercise into your daily routine. The lower the number, the more you need to practise the preceding technique. You can also listen to the mind-programming CD that comes with this book as often as you like. The more you listen, the more motivated to exercise you will become.

It's important to remember that no matter how much you want to change, it will still only happen one day at a time. You don't need to start a formal exercise programme (unless you want to clear up your skin, be less moody, and have better sex), but you do need to move your body. Do it whenever you get the chance. Take the stairs instead of the lift. Park further away from the office and walk 2,000 extra steps to work. Move. Dance. Play sports. Have fun. You only have one body, so you might as well enjoy it!

Gillian Todd Hunter
LOST 2½ STONE

BEFORE   **AFTER**

In 1999 my weight had increased to 11st 3lbs. I felt lethargic, my concentration was poor and my physical size caused me to lose my self-esteem. It was time for action. After many failed diets I tried the strict regime of Weight Watchers. The target weight was reached but unfortunately my thought was always food and the weight piled back on until I reached my heaviest weight ever of over 12 stone.

I bought Paul McKenna's Easy Weight Loss CDs. Once I started to listen to the CD in the comfort of our home it quickly filled me with the positive will-power to change my attitude towards food and my body. There were techniques that could be learned, which gave me a different approach to losing weight and staying slim that I had never before considered. It showed me how to understand the signals my body sends me as I eat and how to stop eating when I have had enough. The weight very quickly and easily started to disappear and soon I had reached my target of 10 stone, but much more, I stayed there!

Four years on and I am still 10 stone; I don't have to think about my weight or dieting and food/eating is no longer my every thought. During the last four years I have found with the audio-tape programme that it is simplicity itself. Old eating habits have been replaced, I am now a vegetarian and my new-formed confidence from this positive way of handling my weight has seen me change my job and the way I exercise. This new confidence, which has come from not having to worry about my body size, has helped me become a person with a positive outlook to my life.

Gillian Todd Hunter

CHAPTER SIX

•

Craving Busters

How to take control of your cravings

If you have ever had a craving, you know that it felt like it needed to be satisfied immediately. In addition, most cravings are for a specific food, like chocolate, pizza or cheesecake. Here's all you need to know:

'Paul's system has changed me. I have not eaten chocolate since I started using it.'

ELAINE HOPKINS,
ADMINISTRATOR

**Any craving you may have felt is a
learned behaviour.**

That means you weren't born with it and if you learned it, you can unlearn it, often in a matter of minutes.

There are two techniques in this chapter. If you are in the midst of a food craving, I'm about to share with you a startlingly simple way you can reduce or even eliminate that craving in less than two minutes. If you would like to re-programme your mind to stop a particular craving for ever, you can skip ahead to the second technique . . .

CRAVING BUSTER – NUMBER ONE
TAPPING INTO THE THIN WITHIN

If you are feeling a strong craving now and you want to reduce it immediately, just follow my instructions completely and your craving will vanish. It will seem like magic, but in fact, it's hard science.

What we are about to do involves tapping on certain acupuncture points on your body. This amazing technique was developed by Dr Roger Callahan, author of *Tapping in to the Health Within*. Each of these points controls the flow of energy in your body. By tapping on each point in exactly the sequence I am going to describe, you will be able to control your craving and get on with your life.

This process may seem a bit strange at first, but it works. You will need to be able to really concentrate for a few minutes, as it is important that you continue thinking about the food you have chosen as you go through this process and reduce the craving.

CRAVING BUSTER – NUMBER ONE

Before you do this exercise read through all the steps first.

1. Focus on your craving for a moment. Now, rate your craving on a scale of 1 to 10, with 1 being the lowest and 10 the highest. This is important, because in a moment we want to know how much you've reduced it.

    So think about the food you are craving. On a scale of 1 to 10, how strong is your craving?

2. Continue to think about that food you have been craving and taking two fingers of either hand, tap about ten times firmly under each eye.

3. Now, tap under your collarbone.

4. Keep thinking about the food you were craving and tap under your armpit.

5. Now place your other hand in front of you and tap on the back of it between your ring finger and your pinkie.

Cont …

6. Open your eyes – now close them.

7. Keep tapping, open your eyes, and look down to the right and down to the left.

8. Keep tapping and rotate your eyes round 360 degrees clockwise, and now 360 degrees anti-clockwise.

9. Still thinking about the food you were craving, hum the first few lines of 'Happy Birthday' out loud.

10. Now count out loud from 1 to 5 (1, 2, 3, 4, 5).

11. Now once again hum the first few lines of 'Happy Birthday' out loud.

12. Repeat the beginning of the sequence. Still thinking about the food you were craving, tap under each eye about ten times.

13. Now, tap under your collarbone.

14. Now tap under your armpit.

OK, let's stop and check – on a scale from 1 to 10, what number is your craving at now?

If it hasn't completely gone yet, simply go back through the entire sequence again until it does. It may take as many as two or even three times before you have completely eliminated the craving, although most people report getting their craving down to a manageable level on their first or second try.

By now, your craving is almost certainly down to a manageable level. It may even be gone completely. If it ever comes back, you can simply repeat this process as often as you like, or go through the 'compulsion buster' to re-programme your craving away for ever!

'It's amazing. I can honestly say that I have not eaten chocolate since I started using Paul's system. Prior to that I was eating ten bars a day!

GILL MITCHELL, SOCIAL WORKER

CRAVING BUSTER – NUMBER TWO

On television and in my seminars I do a demonstration where I help somebody who is a chocolate addict become unwilling to eat chocolate ever again – in less than two minutes!

I am now going to show you how to do the same thing for yourself – how you can stop yourself from ever wanting to eat a particular food again. Most people choose chocolate, bread, cookies or some other 'treat' food that has turned from an occasional treat to uplift your spirits to a heavy anchor around your hips and thighs.

(Remember, only do this next technique if you genuinely want to stop eating a particular food for good! If you just want to reduce your craving, go back to 'Tapping into the Thin Within'. Read through this technique in its entirety before you do it.)

CRAVING BUSTER – NUMBER TWO

Before you do this exercise read through all the steps first.

1. Think of a food that you hate – one that really disgusts you. (A woman on one of my trainings who swore that she loved to eat everything finally agreed that she found the idea of eating a plate of human hair repulsive.)

2. Next, I want you to vividly imagine there is a big plate of the food you hate in front of you. Now imagine smelling and then eating the food that you hate, as you squeeze the thumb and little finger of either hand together.

   Really imagine the texture of it on your mouth as you squeeze your thumb and little finger together. Imagine the taste of it, squeezing your thumb and little finger together until you feel utterly revolted.

   When you are feeling a bit nauseous, stop and relax your fingers.

   Cont…

3. Next, I want you to think of the food that you are going to stop eating. When you think of it, notice that you can imagine what a plate of it looks like.

4. Now, make that picture of the food you like bigger, bigger and brighter. Make it huge, until it's bigger than you, and make it even bigger than that. Continue making it bigger and bigger and bring it closer and closer and then pass it through you and out the other side. (Most people say that it feels a bit weird to pass the picture through your body – like when a ghost passes through your body in the Harry Potter stories.)

5. Ready? Squeeze your thumb and finger together and remember the taste of the food you hate, while at the same time imagining eating some of the food you like. Now, imagine the food you like is mixed in with the food you hate.

   Imagine eating the two foods together, the food you love and the food you hate. Keep imagining the taste and texture of the two together. Keep eating them in your mind, a big plate, swallow them down, as you squeeze your thumb and little finger together. That's it, eat even more, more and more until you can't eat any more, then stop.

Cont…

6. Now, think about the food you used to like and notice how it's different now.

You can repeat this process as often as you like until you have completely eliminated your desire for that particular food. You will no longer be a slave to your cravings.

CHAPTER SEVEN

•

Frequently Asked Questions About the Simplest Weight-Loss System in the World™

Here are some of the most frequently asked questions that arise when people start putting this system into practice. If you don't find your questions answered here, you are always welcome to e-mail us or join us on one of our live one-day seminars around the country . . .

This all sounds too simple. Does it *really* work?
Yes!

What if I'm really overweight – can I still use this system or do I need to diet first?
Let me put it very clearly – it's diets and the dieting mentality that was making and keeping you overweight in the first place! When you really look at the evidence of the impact of diets on obesity, it makes you wonder how the people who pitch them can keep a straight face.

I'll say it one more time: *Anything or anyone who tries to tell you what, where, when, or how much to eat is teaching you to ignore your body – and if you're overweight, your body is trying to tell you it doesn't like being ignored!*

I don't care how much you weigh, if you've been overweight all your life, or if all your family are overweight – as you use this system you will lose weight, feel more in control and better about yourself.

It's a huge relief to eat when I'm hungry, but I feel guilty eating whatever I want. Can I do one without the other?
No, no, no, no and no. One of the worst consequences of

the diet conspiracy is that serial dieters are continually looking over their shoulders for the food police, lest they be caught enjoying food and sent back to starvation purgatory. Your body was made to run on food, and it will always tell you what it needs once you learn to listen.

Every time you eat something you don't really want, you're reinforcing the idea that someone other than you and your body knows best about what you need – and whilst that's great news for the advertising industry, it's a recipe for disaster when it comes to losing weight.

I can't seem to quit the clean plate club no matter how hard I try – do you have any further suggestions?
It sounds as though you are still trying to 'will-power' yourself thin, which is a bit like trying to hammer in nails with nothing but a screwdriver. It's not that it's not a useful tool, but rather that it's the wrong tool for the job at hand. By using your imagination instead of your will, you'll find it nearly effortless to leave food on your plate and out of your stomach.

If you're really stuck, try this – cut off a few bites of food before you start eating and either throw them away or sweep them on to a spare plate. Then you can eat everything that's left on your plate (providing you're actually hungry).

It's been nearly a week and I haven't lost any weight yet. What am I doing wrong?

Do you mean besides the fact that you're weighing your-self before the first two weeks are up?

There's an old story about a farmer who gave his daughter a packet of seeds to plant so that she would learn about the natural order of planting and nurturing what you most want to see develop and grow. Yet even though he had given her some of the simplest growing seeds available, nothing new ever seemed to emerge from the field.

One day, the farmer noticed his daughter digging up the seeds and holding them up to the light. When he asked her what she was doing, she told him she had wanted to see if there was anything growing yet. What she didn't realize was that each time she dug up a seed, she was preventing it from evolving at its natural pace.

In the same way, if you keep weighing yourself with-out allowing time for these seeds to take root in your unconscious, the only things that will grow are your stomach, hips and thighs.

What do I do if I fall off the wagon?

It's perfectly OK to make mistakes. As a baby did you walk on your first attempt? When you learned to ride a bike did you wobble at first and come off a few times? Have the world's greatest achievers made mistakes on their journeys to success?

I would assume that in the first few weeks it's highly likely you will have a slip and over-eat, or temporarily forget to follow the rules. It's fine, just return to following the rules again. Some people use a little slip to beat themselves up and tell themselves that once again they have failed; they console themselves with a binge or just give up on the system, resigned to the fact that they will always be fat.

Not this time! Simply go back to following the rules, eat when you are hungry, enjoy each mouthful and when you suspect you are full, stop!

What do I do if I want to binge?

As some of the old patterns of over-eating dissipate, it is not unusual for the odd craving to arise. When it does, proceed directly to the Craving Busters chapter and tap, tap, tap it away!

But what if I am hungry all the time?

Nobody eats all the time; for example, very few people eat on the toilet or while sleeping. The problem is that over years of telling your body what to eat and when, your body has learned that if it doesn't tell you it's hungry, you might starve it. You need to reassure the body that from now on, whenever it needs food that food will be made available to it. You do that by eating when you are hungry (and stopping when you think you're full).

If you're really worried about it, remember to drink a glass of water first (see Chapter Two) or tune in to your feelings and give yourself some love and approval (see Chapter Four).

What if I can't tell when I am full?

In his book *Achieving Vibrance*, Gay Hendricks teaches about a mechanism in the body he calls 'the V spot', which is located in your solar plexus, just below your ribcage and towards the centre of your body. This is actually a muscle that is designed to control the flow of food to the stomach. Unfortunately, it's not a very strong muscle for most of us! However, as you get more and more sensitive to your body's signals, you can actually feel the V spot close off when your body has had enough food.

In the meantime, just stop if you suspect you might be full, knowing that it doesn't matter if you're wrong – you can always start eating again if it turns out your body is still hungry.

What if I drink a lot?

You're not fat because of what you drink – after all, there are plenty of thin alcoholics. The real issue with excessive drinking isn't weight gain, it's unconsciousness – and I'm not talking about drinking until you pass out!

Most people drink so that they don't have to deal with what's really going on in their lives – but now that you've begun this programme, what's really going on in your life is a process of continual, positive change. I would suggest that, at least at first, you don't drink when you eat and don't eat when you are drinking, but if you do, just make sure to continue to follow the four golden rules of the system.

(By the way, if you think you've got a drinking problem, it's best to get professional help – it really can change your life!)

Can I lose weight without any exercise?
Absolutely – remember Chapter Five. It's virtually impossible not to exercise unless you're completely bedridden. (And even then you're probably breathing . . .) My only question for you is, given how easy it is to accelerate your weight loss by moving just a little bit more than you already do, why would you want to lose weight the slower way?

If I exercise more, will I lose weight faster?
I have noticed that when some people reach the desperation point where they decide they 'have to lose weight immediately', they begin starving themselves, power walking, and going to the gym all on the same day. When these people don't lose weight immediately (because they are driving their body into survival mode), they decide that it's all too much and they give up on the whole project.

Any task can be achieved if it's broken down into small enough chunks. That's why it's a good idea to choose a type and amount of exercise that you can succeed at easily and then increase it bit by bit each week. That way, you get to feel in control every step of the way.

Once you've succeeded the first three times, you'll continue doing it for life!

How well does this work? I want to look like the models in magazines . . .

So do the models in the magazines. Most of the pictures you see on magazine covers have been digitally altered in order to make them striking so that you will buy them. It is not representative of reality. Rather than compare yourself to something that doesn't exist it's far better to compare yourself to yourself. Far too many women compare themselves with an airbrushed picture of an anorexic girl on a magazine cover and decide they aren't good enough as a human being. You are likely to feel significantly better if you ask yourself this question instead:

How much better am I getting?

Actually, I lived in New York for a number of years and had the opportunity to meet many of the world's most famous models. What struck me was that even though many of these women looked so incredibly beautiful, they were pretty miserable, which I suppose is understandable given that they're so hungry all the time! I realized that they spent all their time looking for flaws and rarely saw the perfection of who they already were.

As the great philosopher Goethe said, 'It's not so important where we stand, but the direction in which we are moving.' Human beings are usually at any time either getting better or getting worse. If you are getting better, excellent. If you are getting worse, then you know the direction in which you need to move.

The system is working great, but I'm worried that it will stop. What can I do to make sure it keeps working?
It's important for you to realize that the system isn't working – it's you who's working, perfectly. And all you need to do is eat when you're hungry, eat what you want (not what you think you should), eat consciously and enjoy every mouthful, and stop when you think you're full.

Your body is amazing, and the more you trust yourself, the better you will continue to look and feel.

Leaving food on my plate seems such a waste – couldn't I just take smaller portions?
You could, but you'll lose weight quicker if you stop listening to your plate and start listening to your body about how much to eat. Think of it this way – once the food is on the plate, it's already 'wasted'. If you're really concerned about it, save the rest for the next time you eat!

I started losing weight, but now it's stopped. What do I do?
1. Are you eating whenever you're hungry?
2. Are you eating what you actually want, not what you think you should?

3. Are you eating consciously and enjoying every mouth-ful?
4. Are you stopping when you think you're full (even if there's still food on your plate)?

If you can honestly answer yes to each of these questions, then the secret is to *slow your eating speed down even more!*

Here's how it works: your stomach expands and contracts according to how much food you put into it. In the past, you were eating so fast you couldn't hear your body's full signal. Consequently, you overate and expanded your stomach, thereby creating a need for more food to make you full. When you began to slow down your eating speed, you became conscious of what you were eating as you were eating it and were able to notice the full signal much quicker. You ate less food, your stomach contracted, and you needed less and less food to become full.

However, our bodies are highly adaptive. By now, you may have become so used to eating at your new, slower speed that you have once again gone unconscious about what's going on with your body as you eat. By slowing down even more, you will once again 'trick yourself awake', and be able to once again tune in to your body's satiation signals.

A FINAL NOTE

We are at the end of the book – and the beginning of a life where you are in control of your body and what you do (and don't!) put in it.

Remember, there are only four things you need to do to be thin for life:

1. Eat whenever you're hungry.

2. Eat what you want, not what you think you should.

3. Eat consciously and enjoy every mouthful.

4. Stop when you think you're full.

Everything else in the book is here to help – and it will. You don't have to believe it, just follow my instructions. Need some extra motivation? Review Chapter Three and spend some time seeing yourself slim. Finding yourself in an eating frenzy? Review the information in Chapter Four on emotional eating or if it's more urgent go straight to the Craving Buster and tap your troubles away.

Perhaps the most important resource you have is the

mind-programming CD which I have created to assist you in making what used to be difficult changes easy and enjoyable. Play it every day to reinforce the positive changes you have already begun to make.

Remember, I can make you thin – but it's up to you to take the simple daily actions that will make being thin a habit – and some habits were made to last a lifetime!

Until we meet,
Paul McKenna